YOU, YOUR BEDROOM & 5 MINUTES

SUNIL MIMANI

Become
Shakespeare
.com

First published in 2015 by

BecomeShakespeare.com
Wordit Content Design & Editing Services Pvt Ltd
Newbridge Business Centre, C38/39,
Parinee Crescenzo Building, G Block,
Bandra Kurla Complex, Bandra East,
Mumbai 400 051, India
T: 91 22 33040620

ISBN 978-93-83952-26-7

at-once

one of the juiciest & loftiest non-fiction cver written

CONTENTS

PREFACE

since *Only* pregnant women have *real* justification to the pot-belly,
aren't *other* pot-bellies sheer manifestation of laxity?

Regardless...   we all tend to preserve *this* tendency to acquire *the-belly*.

There is *this* belting-muscle *Transverse*, in the tummy.
Job-its it is, to keep the tummy-&-the-trunk toned.

But because it wouldn't engineer body-movements, the Transverse's role in the body system goes ridiculously-unsung.

Leaving it to perennial-disuse.

And muscles are either *used or ..losed* !

Once the Transverse is lost though,
not only does the belly loose-off its tone,

but also does it start layering-up the superfluous-fat that a toned Transverse should have been burning-off.

now Whilst the layered-fat does get occasionally addressed through diets, workouts & liposuctions, the primary issue of training-toning the Transverse gets more-often-than-not sidelined...

..as much by regular-gymmers & athelets, as by weight-loss-enthusiasts.

becoming indeed,
the precise reason why 'well-built gymmers-&-athelets *with* pot-bellyish-tummies' aren't exactly the exceptionality one would have expected them to be.

It was **indeed** the case of these 'well-built people with weak-Transverse' *that* set my 'physiological-mind' into devising *something* that would keep the *tummy toned **as a matter of routine***.

Glad to have engineered what I like to call *AbChestration*!
Relaxing-&-Healing *to the core*, you would love to call it **EnjoyChestration**.

but could any journey-to-gold ever be easy ?

The innocuous seeming mission proved to be as complex as it could!

as one went about the job, there **kept** emerging *subjective-nuances begging objective-conciliation* !

Pinning-down the technically-correct possibilities couldn't have gotten tougher.

..and given the *fleeting-subtelities* involved, selecting the best amongst them *had* to be hair-splittingly close!

Took no less than a tumultuous 4yrs of painstaking research-&-validation to skim out the dismayingly-close *variants*, and engineer AbChestration to be the very-most valuable that it could be.

So what you finally get is an utterly *game-changing-protocol* that keeps you **tummy-toned** over as much as **an-entire-lifetime**!

..& could you ask for more.. if it came *At* a *P*rice as-sheer-as **5 bedroom-minutes mere.**

Happy reading!
Sunil mimani

Happened to enter the planet back in the 50s...

Birthing mediocre & staying that way for 3decades....
In the 6th decade still generally mediocre.

But...With this *angle of exception* in what could be called mindful-intellectuality.

...

so shan't be it pondered what could have brought this about ?
..what is it that *drives* ?
& indeed what is it, that *sustains* one's intellectuality?...

Whilst thinking-propensity *has* to be the source
of all intellectuality,
and open-mindedness its driving-fuel,
whatever sustains intellect, cannot but *must have
to* hinge upon one's *core-fitness.*

To be sure, I have more than my share of
deficiencies & debilities...

&Yet.. not only do I live,
but do so intellectually.
And,
sustainedly so!

because
I have a trained *core* backing-up my body-brain
system.

The logic of *'body-core **pivotality'*** to the body-mind system remains plain.
And yet we, docs-coaches-&-all included, treat it as nobody's-business!

I am neither a doc, nor a coach.
...Just that deep thinking physiology-scientist, who decided to traverse this *unwalked path*

To construct-&-*culture* this **utmost core-fitness-strategy** for the *thinking* men-&-women of the modern-era.

So go ahead, …but don't *just* enjoy *the–read* !

…take the time to learn & ***instill*** this science of..

core-fitness.

for-a-lifetime.

...

"but then.. Where exactly is this *body-core?*"

Body-Core?... Where & What?

since the context has to be *human-structurality*, what-much would straight away come-through is that *the core has to be somewhere in the body's central-trunk-region*.

But because stopping at the central-trunk wouldn't serve much *actional-purpose*, shouldn't we be trying to close-in & progress towards isolating-out the *actionably-powerising* components of the central-trunk.

And to do so,
shan't the progression be run through a *mechano-metabolic*-comb-up of the central-trunk bones, ligaments & muscles...

and if you did that, what would you expect to find?
One finds that whilst in conformity with anticipation, *the bones & the ligaments* form the trunk's-*structural-framework*
& the *gross muscles* make up the trunk's-*movement-machinery*,

these components being primarily *local* in their functionalities, hardly possess specific *systemic*-attributes that could lead to the body's-*physiological-powerising!*

So what would remain *then* in the central-trunk to comprise the body's *core-powerising-system* ?

by sheer elimination, the *core's-powerising-system* must then comprise of those *innermost tummy-back-muscles*,
that owing to the technicality of their *non-movementality*[1], go ignored over lifetimes-together !

And as of-course irony would have it, they happen to be the *precisely* those that are the *most crucial* in sustaining the core's form-&-firmity.

Which Ones ? ...   I could hear you ask.

---

[1]   *non-causing* of body-movements.

Well, they are your:

> ➤ ***Levators & Coccygei,*** the muscles lying at the *tummy-**base***, in the ***ano-pee-axis***, the medico's *perineum* -
> that happens to be the stretch from the *anus to the pee-outlet.*
>
> *&*

> ➤ The belting-muscle ***Transverse,***
> that happens to be the ab-musculature's innermost-layer that *circles the-tummy- &-the-back* like a ***belting***!

Contrastingly, the outer 6pack-muscle lies in layers outer to the transverse-belting, and is important in its own right, and therefore be indeed exercised-&-built with bending-crunching-exercises.

Just that,
that should happen over & **above a wholesome-core** of the inner belting-&-base.

...if not for the *physical-reason* of being at the body's-structural-base, then for the *physiological-*

reason of being at the centre of body-functionalities as crucial as the *evacuatorial-regulation* of the poo & the pee lines,

to

the modulation-of.. *metabolism,* the very *chemistry of livingness* !

Isn't straight then, that regardless of all exercise, the body's belting-&-base *too* deserve to be worked-out *in specificity*!
...if only to keep the *core-itself* in good form-&-functionality.

..another story, that in addition to conditioning the core-itself,
these work-outs also fortify *this* body-stabilizing *belting-reflex*[2] that integrates peripheral-movements to the body-core.

And doesn't all of *this* add up to *that* compelling-cause to loop-in a *core-specific-program* into one's living ?

---

[2]   *Transverse-Belting*'s reflex-activation in anticipation of body-movement.

May be…
But then, what with the exercise, swimming, gym-ing, athlete-ing and what not *alls* to be done,
where indeed is the time to work the base-&-the-belting ?

YY5 brings to you this **life-changing-protocol** to work the *core-est of your cores* **in** less than **5minutes-a-day** !
&
In a manner, that not only do the *same 5mins* also double-up as a *body-relaxing-rest*, but even triple-up as a *mind-relaxing-meditation.*

Could you have asked for more ?

Mustn't you,
Simply *have to*,
Read on ….

Lights, Camera, Action

Lie there down…
In *anywhich* manner that would comfort your body.

and Even whilst the sideways-curled-position is amongst the more conducive ones,

the best option would be to lie-down in a manner that goes with the *moment's comfort-ambiance.*

And yes,   not on some yoga-mat-type,
but on a proper mattress-&-pillow !

..because,   whilst **AbChestrating**,   you'd have to be *actually* relaxing !

...

Yes...   *AbChestration*!

because *this* workout is *that* construct of working *those* abs in *that* orchestrational-sequence!

...

regardless, I expect you to be lying-down-comfortably by now.

and, if so,

little harm in shutting-off those beautiful eyes as well!

And yes, keep repeatedly changing posture-&-position during the workout

to

whatever comfort-ambiance would prompt you to.

...

in the meanwhile

Let a friend be reading-out this segment, as you practice for the first few days.

Relax.

yes relax

In the eye-shut-lying-down position for-a-while, and then.. when you feel relaxed, focus on your breath for a moment.

Realize that rather than being a deep-breathing-exercise, *AbChestration* is an orchestration of tummy-movements with <u>regular-breathings</u>.

So keep breathing relaxedly for a while
& then.. when you feel-like starting,

relax the tummy & **pull-in a random breath,**

_____

& then

_____

1. pulling the navel in, **execute an exhale** *(*with pauses & holds, *as-urged)* that is **driven by the navel-pull-in.**
Till... after all pauses-&-holds, **the exhale** *melts* **into inhalation.**

2. **breathe-in**...with its pauses-&-holds, *expanding-the-tummy* & *pulling-the ano-pee-axis upwards for a moment.*
Till, after all pauses-&-holds, **the inhale** *melts* **into exhalation.**

3. **execute the exhale**... **navel-driven-ly,** with all its pauses-&-holds,
Till it melts into inhalation.

4. **execute the inhale** *pulling-up the ano-pee-axis momentarily,* & *expanding-the-tummy.*
Till, the inhale with all its pauses-&-holds, **melts into exhalation**

& so forth...
for <u>whatever</u> *would* **feel** *like a span of 5mins.*

And lo.. you're done for the day!

..even if the span clocked no more than
1.5 minutes.
&
even if the breaths felt *labored*, *shallow*, *staggered*
& *overlapped*.

...
All is well, as long as even the subtlest of tummy-
movements happen ed!

& even whilst all you do is keep breathing in the *moment's-flow*, with corresponding tummy movements,

know that the best way to implement *AbChestration*

is to keep it *light* during the initial-minute, raise it to a *moderate* level in the middle-minute, & then *taper* it off during the final-minute.

Though, being about the moment's flow, *AbChestration* will tend to get executed a little differently on different days.

Take all such in your stride, as long as the smallest-&-the-subtlest of accompanying tummy-movements happen!

also Know, that owing to the body's continuously fluctuating metabolic ambiance, breath-lengths could be as dramatically varied as, certain ones being only a fraction of their counterparts!

So that, not only could *AbChestration* get executed a little differently on different occasions, AbChestrational-breaths within the same session too, could be relatively long, short, fast or slow, depending upon the body's *micro-metabolic-ambiance* of the moment.

Know also, that the *upward-pull of the ano-pee-axis during the breathe-in-phase,* is a *keggal-value-addition*[3] that could be dispensed with, whenever breathing-in tends to feel difficult with the upward-pull.

..you'll still reap the core-rewards of AbChestration,

& could always do 'breath-independent-Keggals' at another time!

In other words, do the 'ano-pee-axis pull-ups' only on occasions they would work.

On other occasions, simply carry on with AbChestration without the breathing-in's *base-upping*.

---

[3]   named after the inventor Dr. Keggel, the *kegall-exersice* entails **ano-pee-axis pull-ups** to *work* Levators-&-Coccygei, *the base-muscles.*

The first few sessions nonetheless could be a little *mixing & non-happening*:

Synchronizations would come through though earlier than anticipations. So rather than giving up, keep at applying moderate *navel-inning-&-base-upping* effort during those *spontaneously-lengthed*-breathing-phases.

To be sure, moderate power application is at-once ample-&-optimum for the revival & sustenance of those hitherto neglected muscles!

Nevertheless.. once the navel-inning & base-upping sequences-&-synchronizations come through, one might occasionally like to apply full-muscle-contraction-&-hold.

but yes... <u>Occasionally Only</u>, please!

As I said, on a day to day basis, **moderate**-muscle-force **abchestration** is the one that is **optimum** in sustaining physio-structural-firmity.

Moving to *Mind-ities*!

...to *deduce-out* the AbChestrational *medito-relaxacity*.

Don't we begin with zeroing-in on the core of *all meditationality*?

Well... whichever way you research & look at the abounding systems of meditational-forms, you'll find that the *only essentialities* they have in-common *are*, that they all aim to:

steady, calm & relax
the wandering, panicked & the taxed mind.

Juxtaposing this '*steadying-calming meditational-essentiality*'with the AbChestrationally *synchronized-breathing-system* :

Could the mind help getting *reigned-in* for those 5mins.? ...
& Wouldn't therefore, the mind's-
wander stop...panic melt.. & taxedness ease.

& Hadn't so, you had moved towards steadiness, calmness & relaxedness ?

And if you had,
Hadn't you *had* already *abchestro-meditated* ?

Dive back into physicalities!

Transcending back to the physicalities of *breathing length-&-pace*, time now to calibrate the *inaptness of over-breathing* to perspective.

Beginning-with & *basing-on* the background-science of Breathing's *driving-role* in cellular-metabolism,

over-&-under-breathing-notions ought to be reckoned *in-relativity* to the body's *metabolic-currency*.

Ranging from being in complete-rest, to say, being in a volatile-soccer-session !

So that, whilst in the heightened-metabolic-state of the soccer-session, rapid-&-over-breathing is apt,

in the resting-metabolic-state, quite-&-slow breathing is indeed the best.

Because...

owing to the physiological-technicalities of *vasoconstriction*[4] & *bohr-effect*[5], **over-breathing** actually, even if *so-paradoxically*, leads to **under-oxygenation**! of the body-&-the-brain.

And so if you sense overbreathing in an AbChestrational-Session, either be able to reduce the overall-breathing-volume,
or else

cut-out & abort the process *then*,
to do it another time again !

---

[4] **overbreathing-spurred** narrowing of blood-tubes, leading to **lowering of oxygenation** in the brain-&-the-body.

[5] **overbreathing-spurred** fall in *breathen-oxygen*'s transfer-to-tissues, *also* leading to **oxygenation-lowering** in the brain-&-the-body.

Before you ask...

A few more *significancies* to be noted right away:

I. AbChestration is meant to be done during free-time, when one could afford to relax.
Since it could interfere with external-focus, *AbChestration* is best <u>avoided</u> during attention-intensive-activities like <u>driving & swimming</u>.
& for that matter, why just driving & swimming? *AbChestration* is best avoided during all real-time-activities at all !

Unlike AbChestration though, momentary *abbings* (as you'll get to know in a fortnight's time), could be done to-advantage in all scenarios of real-time-activity.

II. Whilst *AbChestration* could be gainfully done twice-a-day, **once** in a day is **good** enough.

And as long as a 5minutes eye-shut-lying-down is possible,

any non-tasking-time from breakfast to supper is *good*,

so long as one is not in a tired, sleepy *or such*-state.

III. Even whilst AbChestrational-practice does not warrant lifestyle-changes, the practice of *sundry-breathing-exercises* of whatever names-&-description, would best get *cut-out*…even if for a mere fortnight.

So that you steer clear of fouling-up your abchestrational-synchronizations.

& in any case, *there isn't one breathing-benefit that AbChestration doesn't confer* !

IV. Tried to practice *AbChestration*, but *doesn't happen* only?

Most of the time this happens when one tries to force-elongate or force-complete one's breathe-ins or breathe-outs:

Breathe long only if that is happening spontaneously.

Not only is *uneven-&-short-breathing synced AbChestration* fine, it is optimum as well.

Also know that rather than being a *micro-precision*, AbChestration is more of an *overall-pattern*. So that, frequent unevenness-overlaps-&-such, are all part of the game. All's well though, as long as even the subtlest of tummy-movement is happening.

so don't over-exert-&-over-perfectionise.
Simply prefer a *light*, **relaxed** *& playful* execution-of-abchestration.

V. Why should abchestration be done lying-down? Why not sitting, standing & walking?

Whilst abChestration is technically *do-able* in all postures-&-positions, I would commend the comfortable lying-down-posture, **so** that one is in a perfect position to extract-out the *triple-mileage* of 'core-work-out, *body-relaxation & relaxo- meditation'*
from within those **same** *5minutes*.

...

For the standing-up & sitting-down positions, there are variations that I'll let you know in the next segment!

The next segment though is better read after getting a hold of the basic abchestrational synchronization.

Around a fortnight's-practice, generally.

So, bye for now.. until we meet again after your 1st-fortnight of *AbChestration*.

But we meet with the precondition that you start the book all over again & reach here all over again,   even if in jet-speed...

Just so to make sure that the *powerising-algorithm* links-&-sums-up *just* right.

The Abbing-Chestration(al) system

So you have been practicing abchestration through the fortnight..

Did you notice that besides enhancing body-tone, abchestration also does that big plus to your energy-levels!
This happens because whilst working-out those core-abs, *AbChestration* is *also* silently *working-out* one's core-*metabolism*, that *core-chemicality of all live-energy*.

So how about *this* happening *through-the-day*?
How about practicing abchestration sitting, standing & walking?
Might sound good, but bad-idea really.

Bad idea
because being absorbing, abchestrational-indulgence could distract one *out* from *realtime-living*,
& therefore, could increase *physical-mishaps* potentiality.

"O.K.   If *mishaps happen,   we'll tackle!*"

Good *Spirit*!
But *should* that be goading one to *knowingly* invite-&-invoke the *ever willing planetary-mishaps*?

AbChestration must therefore be *mandatorily* **restricted to** *mishap-proof-situations* of a level where one could *safely* chance to *lie-down-in-shut-eyes*: the so named *'eye-shut-lying-down' -tolerant* **scenarios.**

But then, since it is physiologically advantageous to garner the wholesomeness of abchestrational *diaphragmatic-continuum*[6] all through, **YY5** has built-up this technique of **abbing-chestration,** to possibilise *all-scenario-powerising* without having anything to do with those *ever-willing* planetary mishaps.

To understand **abbing-chestration** though, one would rather first practice-out what is best called **abbing!**

---

[6]   the state in which one's predominant *breathing-mode* is **diaphragmatic,** rather than the relatively inefficient *chest-breathing mode.*

Abbing

"Is the technique of *triggering-up* the body's *subliminal ab-chestrationality* at-will"

So aligned is abchestration to physiological-nuances, that once *into it*, the body tends to continue the process autonomously, even-if *subliminally*.

year-on-year of indifference, if not downright reverse-conditioning, succeeds nevertheless in engineering a quick petering-out!

Given a *trigger* though, the body would tend to *restore* the *subliminal-abchestrationality*, even if for a bit.

So how about triggering-up the process every some-while?
Wouldn't the body get into a *functional-flow* of *abchestrational-wholesomeness* ?

Abbing was purpose-designed to deliver this-very!

And, what do you do, *to do the abbing*?
Precious-little, really.

All you need *do*
is to :

"momentarily **tuck that navel IN a little-bit**, and
then forget !"

You *already* did an **abb-in**!

Do it in *random-periodicity*, do it to address
boredom-&-laxity, do it for *athletic-priming-posturing*,
..do it *wherever-whenever*!

And yes, the tuck-in needs to be very subtle only,
so you could do it *sub-semi consciously*, without
getting out of the present.

The same result of abchestrational-triggering
could also be reached...

If instead of a navel tuck-in, you did a ***momentary base-upping***. And if you did that, you know you did an **abb-up**.

Needless to say, both **abbing-in & abbing-up** would have the same effect of   abchestrational-triggering.

Abbing-in being more intuitive though,   tends to be the default-triggering-mode.

However, on occasions when owing to an *ongoing breathing-in-phase*, abb-in just wouldn't come-through,
or for that matter, on random-occasions as well...
one could simply do that momentary 'abb-up'.

Abbing-in or abbing-up... the key thing to know is that, rather than being about doing the abchestration consciously,
abbing is only about ***just*** triggering it on, & then forgetting!
After all, abbing was purpose-devised to lace you with the capability to reap abchestrational-mileage during the course of the day, without having to tie-up one bit of real-time-consciousness.

Owing to the physiology of *conditioning* though, the abbing-tool would need around a fortnight of abchestrational-practice to get going.

Abbing-Chestration

Could it be anything other than the aggregation of abchestration & abbing ?

Well it certainly is... and some more!

Times and moods happen when even whilst the body tends to abchestrate, the mind's meditationality simply wouldn't come-through!

So what do you do then, *when* even in the absence of the accompanying-meditationality, the body wouldn't still stop abchestrating ?

Well... you *abchestrate*,
pause,
may-be *abb*,
may-be *abchestrate* without base-uppings,
may be *pause* again to moderate-out that bit of overbreathing,
and then *abb* again...
and do the whole thing without any conscious tracking of the breath!

Abbingchestration is indeed a *pausing-peppered* fuzzy-mix of abchestration & abbing!

Little wonder, abchestrational-postgraduates *core-up* a lot of the time *abbingchestringly*.

They are post-grads because they have developed that knack of spontaneously reverting back-&-

forth from *abchestration* to *abbing* to *regular–breathing*, without having to move out of the present.

Whilst one couldn't be doing it right-away, know that abbingchestration does *happen* at some point in one's abchestrational-journey.

Just that.. the *happenance* tends to come-about with this *paradoxical-requirment* of having to *actually* cut-back & **moderate-out** one's abbingchestrational-indulgence!
& *why?*...

Because, doing it all over could lead to risking that chance of occasionally losing control of breathing-balance and regressing into   *metabolically–inapt* over-breathing...

And not only does metabolically inapt over-breathing lead to *that* paradoxical-lowering of brain-body oxygenation,

but could also trigger the *innate–nervous–system*[7] into panic-mode,

leading to all sort of disarray, ranging all the way from *B.P.-jump-slumps* to *gut–misdemeanors*.

& even whilst all of this could be reversed by reversing the metabolically-inapt over-breathing,

---

[7]   is the **un-willable** *component* of the *nervous–system*. Based on *its* perception of the body's internal-&-external environment, it **autonomously** *modulates* the body's-internal-functioning.

best is clearly,
to curb, restrain, avoid & abort abbingchestrational-
indulgence in scenarios of over-breathing!

Abbing, though could be done in such and
whatever kind of scenarios.
In fact, pace-&-length-unrestrained abbingchestration could be advantageously replaced
with sheer *abbing*, that momentary navel-inning
or base-upping without breath-syncing!
Even otherwise, staying s*lightly abbed-in-or-up*
generally is not a bad idea at all !

Also, recall & indeed *re-instill* the concept   that
abbing is a tremendous tool for *athletic-priming-
posturing*.
So *make it in your system* to be generally-abbing
when sporting-exerting-or-exercising.

Abchestration though, is adequate-enough just
once-a-day!

& Abbingchestration ?

Needn't be any more than a couple of short-spells
across the day:

things like those random 2minute-spells or maybe that *one-breath* minispell before coming out of the bed,   &-such.

A Quick Actional-Recap

of the *3As*, ...just so to put things in perspective.

"w*hilst Abchestration is the conscious work-out of the belting-&-the-base,
& Abbing, just that momentary pull-in or pull-up;
Abbing-chestration is their pausing-peppered aggregation, to cater to* spontaneities &-such."

And actionally:

"*whilst **Abbing** is a triggering & posturing-priming tool,
do-able **anytime-anywhere**,*

*& **Abbingchestration** a base-belting mix,
preferably do-able **lying-down, in lieu of abchestration** ;*

Abchestration *is the full-involvement relaxo-meditational work-out,
mandatorily do-able* <u>only</u> **in 'eye-shut-lying-down'-tolerant scenarios.**"

...

But then, since abbingchestration lends itself so well to spontaneities, shouldn't the postgrads simply replace abchestration with abbingchestration?

Well, whilst abbingchestration would sure suffice on a day-to-day basis, even the veterans would need to be occasionally practicing abchestration too,
..if only to keep the *ab-conditioning* going!

&finally...
even whilst the specifics vary,   allow me to *refro-pack* the three as **Ab3.**

Congratulations on your abchestrational degree!

Now that you are well on the way to attaining abchestrational-postgraduation yourself, how does it feel like?

Do you feel happy getting a hold on your physicality. Or do you feel it is all a monetisational-hoax?

Without doubt, I stand to make money every time the book gets bought, but isn't that merely a *commercial-incidentality* of cost-recovery?

"The moving-motive of this book has all-through been formativity."

Nothing else whatsoever was let to impact the work in any manner *whatsoever*.

Know that when it comes to functionality, Ab^3 by virtue of its metabolism modulation-al effect, has an optimisational-impact on every single of the body's-internal-system, right upto the neuro-harmonal-pathways.

And know that when it comes to structurality, not only does the *Ab3-system* tone the tummy, but is also your biggest back-protector, happening as it does, to be the *utmost toner* of your *personal-backbrace* Transverse, the internal-belting!

So why wouldn't you make use of the ab3-system to see your base-&-belting powerise you!

...
Whilst any residual-issues would always be referable to me, let's have at least the obvious ones talked-out upfront:

Docs&Coaches

Why hasn't the Ab³ got backed by the medical & the coaching fraternities or for that matter, so much as even gotten mentioned by the university-academia?

Even whilst *YY5* is intended to be a copyrighted-text, realize that regardless of its genesis as a proprietary-process, **Ab3** would always be positioned as a *trade-&-patents-proof-package*!

Indeed! You are invited to adopt the process and spread the good word!

Coming to the question-proper though, the medical-fraternity has to, of sheer necessity,   be so preoccupied with correctives-&-fixatives, that there remains little time-&-room left for prevention-&-augmentation.

However docs, & in particular the pot-bellied ones amongst you,

I invite you to try the process out on yourselves, if only for just a fortnight !

Ab^3 is purpose-designed for people pressed-for time.

So tone-up the core, relax-up the limbs, and indeed free-up the mind, within those *same* 5minutes.

Or, do you see a hidden-risk, or for that matter, have finally located *that* 'damaging flaw'?

Ab3 being a comprehensively-proofed output of an exhaustive-research, the author in me has the conviction to challenge medical fraternity the world-over, to confront me with *that* most tangential-flaw in the Ab3-system.

I would be happy to clarify, even whilst being sporting-enough to get clarified!

Until then though, rather than being dismissive & procrastinating, start abbing right away, the good doc!

The coaching and the training fraternity tends to be occupied primarily with individual-sport specific moves, and hence concerned primarily with the building of peripheral-and-outer-muscles. That is how their profession must operate, if they were going to be in business! Ab^3 being a new concept, is bound to take some time to sink into the *must-do* list of the coaching-fraternity, but once a few top coaches try it out themselves, the scene cannot but transform overnight !

I invite top coaches & trainers to practice-out Ab³ themselves, to experience its core-conditioning value first-hand.

"So convinced will you all get in just a few weeks, that holding the technique back from your trainees would become an impossibility for **each-one** of you!"

The universities are supposed to be seats of intellectual-pursuits, and I am not saying they aren't, but such importance have monetizationalities & *other-externalities* gained in recent times, that even mainstream universities could be readily spotted straying into downright-nonrighteous-indulgences that could range all the way *from*

endorsing rigged-researches

to

patronizing half-sciences like Homeopathy & Ayurveda

to

legitimizing even complete non-sciences like Astrology & Vaastu !

I recently stumbled into this research team-leader from a globally leading university, admitting out of guilt that the result that they could *get* published in *that* benchmarking-journal was not the *one* that they got 6-times in 7experiments, ..but the *one* that they got *once* in 7experiments!

...for a reason as foul as that of the *rigged-result making the more sell-able story* !!

No, not by any stretch would I want my research to be tagged with a university authentication !

..If a university-team though does get interested in a genuine study of abchestration, the scientist in me would be more than willing to coordinate.

Know though in the meantime that Ab[3] is not some *beta* or -such,

"It is the final-package of a one hundred percent proofed-research."

So do get started the day you finish reading.
& indeed lead the way, the good doc.!

Those 6-pack abs?

Abchestration is neither in competition with,
nor in contradiction to,
other exercises.

So that, even whilst restricting abchestration to
'*eye-shut-lying-down*-compliant scenarios' makes
sense,
abbing could be advantageously integrated-into
all sort of athletical-activity.

And...
One specific workout of particular synergy *is* the
crunch,
in which, **the upper-trunk is *armlessly* lifted
from a legs-folded-lying-down position.**

& the Crunch is the specific 6-pack tool, not Ab3.

Ab3 tones-up the internals & gives you that
toned-tummy, but if you also fancy the cosmetics
of the outer 6pack, crunching needs to be looped-
in too into your system, and it doesn't take rocket-

science to see that any crunching-regimen could only hugely benefit from the **Ab3's** *background-conditioning*.

Crunch or no crunch...
the core reality is that all exercise work way-more-wholesomely with the *reflexive-coring*[8] of Ab[3],
and that much more lopsidedly, when done without the *ab-referencing*.[9]

---

[8] reflexive-anchoring by the belting-base core.
[9] periodic abbing during athletical-activities to keep reflexive-coring primed-up.

Exercises of the *body-peripherals*,[10] when done without *natural-or-learnt* abbing, tend to result in a combination of developed peripheral-muscles **with** a developed-tummy-paunch,
the *combination* being the result of a *skewed regimen sapping-off* as it were, the *belting's base-tone* into the peripherals !

..things wouldn't go that way though, if only the coaches insisted upon exercises being executed *tucked-inly.*

I expect the coaches of the future to actively instruct a *systemic-practice* of the Ab^3 and to be insistent upon all exercising-&-sporting being done *bracedly*... paving the way for that *ideal-combination* of **toned-peripherals-&-toned-abs**!

So what are you waiting for?
Ab^3 is going to be *so synergic* with all your physio-mental endeavors, even whilst being *so sparing* on all your resources.
And..

---

[10]   muscles-&-structures away from the body-center.

with *all those* medito-relaxational *credits* too *bundled-in there* into the deal,

Why-y on the planet wouldn't you get started bang on the day you finish this book?

Beyond Ab3

"Ab3 so good, won't it enable me to do away   with other whole-health systems?"
I am afraid not.

Even whilst firming-up core structurality, revving-up core metabolism & firing-up the core neuro-harmonal-system, Ab^3 is still not pervasive enough to bypass the fundamental *whole-health-systems* of **Rest, Hygiene & Nutrition.**

Here is an *addressive-list* of the more frequently missed *hygo-nutri-essentials*:

I. *Structure* daily-eats to make for that *non-taxing* **MRP-inclusive-nourishment.**

where,

_M_ would be the-
  vite-mineralistic **_M_**_icro-nutrients_ *in:* <u>fruit-
veggie-greens</u>.

_R_ would be the-
  *plant-**R**oughage in:*
<u>fruit-veggie-greens</u>.
  &

_P_ would be the-
  _P__roteins-&-**P**robiotics_[11] *in:*
<u>dairy</u>^{poultry} -<u>legume</u>^{nuts} with <u>curd-yogurt-must</u>.

---

[11] comprising of y..es! edible-organisms, probiotics
work by *fixing* the gut's parasitic-microbes.

  Found randomly in pickled-fermented-edibles... the
most authentic source of probiotics is the 'curd-yogurt'
food-category.

  So that, with all the top-notch protein-content that it
has.., it is still its '*irreplacable probiotic-content*', that raises
'curd-yogurt' to the ultimacy of being: the-most
  un-tradeable *human-food available* on the planet!

Carbs & Fats, if at all, need *negative-targeting* on account of their propensity to creep-in *anyway* into all sort of cuisine.

So ignoring them & going by the *overlap* in **MRP-sources**, all one needs to *automate* that non-taxing *MRP-inclusive-nourishment*, is to: include <u>something daily</u> from each of the 3 "***DFC eat-actional-groups***" consisting of:

D: *dairy-poultry-legume-nuts.*
F: *fruit-veggie-greens.*
C: *curd-yogurt must.*

Indeed,
As long as all *the 3DFC eat-actional-groups* get represented in daily-eats, humans across the globe could count themselves *MRP-nourished.*

So regardless of cuisines & settings, ***vary meals*** to facilitate daily-**inclusions** from all of the 3 **DFC** (<u>dairy-fruit-curd</u>) *eat-actional-groups* & stay ***MRP***-*inclusively*-**nourished** all the way!

Nevertheless, on days when all dietary plans-&-prudence fail, consider popping-in a *vit<u>e</u>-min multi*[12] to compensate for the missed micros, *as also* sipping-up something like the *yakult* probio-drink to make-up for those missed-probios. The delicious *yakult* though could be gainfully had even on the curdy-yogurty-days!

& Yes, replace some of those liver-intensive caffeine-cuppers with the way-more wholesomely-delicious choco-malty *bournvita*! The clincho-quation:

"Toxic–caffeine vs. Nutritious–cocoa!"

Make exceptions though! On occasions when one could access those peerless signature-cuppas at cafes like the *m.t.r.* & the *koshy's* of Bangalore, the coffee-capital of India.

---

[12] multi *vitamin-mineral* supplement.

The wholesomely-delicious *bournvita* though should still deserve the day-to-day prevalence over all the world's best caffeine-cuppas put together!

II. On-the-go *oro-dental-sanitization* :

In addition to the regular-brushings, doing a couple of *drinking-water-rinses*[13] of the <u>side-&-back-teeth</u> after *filming-souring-ingestions*,[14] makes for that oft-skipped *on-the-go oral-sanitization* !

---

[13] commended *drinking-water-rinses* would comprise of **side-&-back-teeth rinsing** with drinking-water-sips, *before swallowing them in*.

[14] are of foods-&-drinks that are either *sticky or sour*. Resultant *tooth-souring-&-filming* warrants early-*wash* in the interest of *tooth-erosion minimization*.

Also handy is the strategy of reserving a few *tooth-cleansing fruit-veggie-chunks*[15] for those final-morsels of the meal.

---

[15]   owing to their roughage-content, fruit-veggies have a general cleansing-effect in the mouth.

Sour-fruit though are better had in the meal's-initial-stages, so that the following meal-courses *auto-wash-off* some of that sourness.

& also so that.. the idea of **desserting** on fruit-veggies be applied to the **non-sour-ones** only.

III. Intend to keep the immune-system on your side!

Since the immune-system is a finite faculty, the <u>case</u> of '*overloadings potentialating into sundry infect o–flammations to, as much as cancer level wrath-menifestations*', <u>stands</u> as much to inductive-rationale, as much does *it stand* to deductive-reasoning.

Why would you risk all that when even whilst being un-*proofable*, the risk could *still* be covered *so much more* through sheer '*informed-segregation*'[16] from the in-&-around microbial-abundance.

..& evenwhilst Cleansers-&-Disinfectants abound, & of-course ought to be used in balance, the following-two on account of their *yet* hugely untapped sanitizational-potential, merit specific-mention.

---

[16] segregation-from, manifest-&-*likely* moldy-rotting surfaces by

(a)keeping safe-distance

&

(b)by practicing *need-based* & *routine-based* washing-disinfecting.

1) The 'hypochlorite-based original-domex', that being laced with exhaustive-germicidal-power, is as-much-assuring for need-based-pourings, as-much-is-it for the routine-ones: *onto* the 'kitchen-toilet-surfaces' & *into* the 'toilet-sink-drains'!

   &

2) The *betadine*-gargle, *that* iodine-based ultimate mouth-throat-disinfectant that goes beyond its place in the medicine-cabinet to deserve a place in the cloakroom-cabinet as well, to promote those *preemptive weekly-rinses...*

And whilst on the subject, I would like to commend this exceptional website for cutting-edge-insights on the immune-system's load-limiting:

http://www.safespaceco.com is an exceptional commercial-website that is more enlightening than many of the academic-websites on the subject!

Ab3 Ir-replaceable!

Transcending back nonetheless to Ab^3:

I. Why shouldn't one simply replace the ab3-system with those off the shelf Orthopedic-Back-Belts?

Whilst external-beltings can be of assistance to the injured-spine, there is no way they can make for the wholesomeness of the real transverse-belting.

Owing to the *eccentric*-tummy-pressurizations they generate, long-period-wearings of external-beltings actually stand to distort the internal-belting's geometry.

Besides, why on planet would one like to avoid working one's own personal-belting, when the workout stands to deliver as much as a *lifetime-of-core-fitness*
at not only
as-less-as 5mins.,

but laced also with the marvel of being so utterly *off-costing-taxing*.

Know that by working the belting & the base in alternation, Ab^3 also relaxes them in alternation. So, much in the manner of the heart-muscle's *self-management-of-fatigue*, Ab^3 too self-manages fatigue through muscle-work-alternation.

"But then does ab3 actually protect the back?"
At the end of the day, as indeed during its course, the only *term-protection* that the human-back can garner, is that of the *transverse- belting's bracedness*.
..and since the entire

Ab^3-system is centered around building-up the transverse's *reflexive-tonality*, Ab^3 cannot but lead to a progressively better-braced & *therefore* a progressively more-protected back.

II. A. Ok, ab3 good, even great, but can't one access the same benefits through the EMS-Systems?
   B. Or through Liposuctional 'tummy-tucks'?

A. EMS-systems work muscles through external electrical-impulses instead of the body's internal nerve-impulses.

To begin with, most of the touted EMS-systems tend to be patently bogus.
There are good Systems though,
but
know first, that since the EMS *bypasses the Nervous-System*, even the best of the

EMS-Systems cannot but have this *vested-inability* to work muscles in the *willed-mode.*[17]

So that, whilst being the *only-option* to work the *uncommandable* involuntary-muscles,
the EMS would deliver *most* to the *commandable* voluntary-muscles, when used <u>in conjunction</u> with *willed-exercise.*

& when it comes to willed-exercise, Ab3 is better there... *right at the core*, in any regimen.

B. Liposuctional tummy-tucks are surgical procedures to effect *mechanical-removal* of fat-deposits.
& whilst they are a good thing to get done for the removal of gross-deposits,
transverse-toning should still be adopted to ward-off subsequent build-ups & to keep the *core* generally *toned-&-tuned* over one's life-span.

---

[17]   is the mode in which muscles can be willed-to-work.
  Whilst most outer-body-muscles can indeed be willed-to-work,
  inner-body-muscles *live* beyond the will's-command & work-solely on the *innate*-nervous-system's signaling.

III. Incontinence has gotten me this prescription for the Keggel-Exercise. Any linkages with abchestration?

Leave-aside linkages,
& be happy to know that the *Ab3* actually embodies the *keggels* in its *breathing-in-phase*!

Know that the celebrated Dr.Keggels' perineal-exercise to condition the ano-pee lines, is exactly the ano-pee-axis pull-up that one does during the abchestrational breathe-in!
So that, even whilst being *ab*preciative of me … do be hugely thankful to Dr.Keggel, the original master of base-upping.

& of course...
in the case of the Keggels being a clinical-priority, it would make sense to be practicing out *abchestration-unsynced-***Keggels** too across the day.

IV. Has abchestration got anything to do with sex and sexuality?

Nothing really!

Abchestration & indeed the whole ab3-complex, is a core-fitness-regime, neutral to sex & sexuality. The odd occasional abbing though   would tend to impart a core-stabilizational-input to the sexing-body!

Tantra-mantra-pranayam and-such!

"Does abchestration relate to mystics & dogmas like the tantra-mantra-pranayam and-such?"

AbChestration is neither a gimmick nor anything dogmatic & has nothing *remotely* to do with occulties & anecdotals.

On the contrary, Ab³ is a painstakingly developed scientific-protocol to form-&-powerise humans across-the-globe.

I. Could abchestration be done whilst eating?

Even whilst abchestration cannot be done during meals, a bit of abbing during *mealing* would definitely go some way in keeping *filledness-signaling*[18] on the edge, helping one keep safe-distance from over-eating.. that villain of all good eating.

II. Should abchestration be done in fatigue? Can abchestration work like a power-snooze?

With all its medito-relaxational attributes, Ab^3 is still a work-out, and work-outs cannot resolve physical-fatigue.

So in conditions of fatigue, it would make sense to first recover with adequate rest. Abbingchestration could always be indulged-into later, when you are better!

Also would go without saying that all abchestration ought to be stopped fore-with in conditions of any sort of body-turmoil, internal or external.

---

[18] from amongst the several-mechanisms *relaying* satiety-signals to the brain, abbing stands to modulate the signaling-of-physical-filledness.

To execute any workout, one first has to be in body-peace, & even then you exert *within the body's-comfort-limits*!

III. Should abchestration be done during pregnancy?

Working the base & the belting *simultaneously* does have the potential to *orient* intra-abdominal-pressure to hazardous-profiles, but the abchestrational-system being woven around *base–belt–**alternation**, studiedly* avoids hazardous-tummy-pressurizations,
making the *Ab3-system* **assuringly pregnancy-safe.**

And so, in the context of the heightened-need-during-pregnancy to stay healthy-&-core-fit, it would make for utter *formative-sense* to continue with one's abchestrational-practice right through one's pregnancy.
Staying within one's comfort-limit though has *historically* **been a great-idea!**

IV. *How* does Ab³ affect poise-&-posture **?**

Since the *spinal-alignment's-aptness or deviance-therefrom*, could be the only plausible-explanation of the human *trunk-al posture*,

& since owing to their unique-anatomical-profile, *the-belting-&-the-base-muscles* happen to be the *prime-regulators* of the *spine's-geometric-alignment*,

& since *the-belting-&-the-base-muscles* sustain their *reflexivity-priming* from learnt-&-innate *Ab3-processes*,

Ab3's posturisational-ity needs no claiming at all !

So do digest & disseminate this bit of a *contrarian-*counsel:

A linear *straight-line-posture* is not a good idea, going as it does, *against* the natural-geometry of the spinal-curvatures...

& so that,
rather than slouching on the one hand,
or getting into a stiff-straight-mode on the other,
simply **lie-sit-stand-&-move**, ***with*** just those ***periodic postural-abbings***.
To be sure, you'd had already *ergo-dynami-sised* !

The way forward!

Well, teach the process to the young-ones just before or during teen-hood:
They will enter & sustain teen-hood that much better.

& of-course, once your kids have their young-ones,
tip *them* to teach it to *their* young-ones,
at *their* threshold-of-teenhood !

"So that the powerising Ab3 percolates–down across generations,
to eventually become a standard–way of human-living!"

bon voyage....
sunil mimani

Glossary

1. AbChestration   : full   involvement medito-relaxational workout of the core.

2. Abbing   : belting's   momentary pull-in or the base's momentary pull-up.

3. AbbingChestration : s e m i - s t r u c t u r e d fuzzy-mix of the two.

* * *

www.ingramcontent.com/pod-product-compliance
Lightning Source LLC
Chambersburg PA
CBHW032118280326
41933CB00009B/890